Tas M

THE REAL-WORLD WEIGHT LOSS BOOK

Dear Person, first of all, thank you for picking this book as your weight loss guide. The reason this book has been written is because I have seen a need to educate people with what they eat in order to lose weight and get themselves healthy. Unfortunately, we live in an age where we are getting fatter and very unhealthy but we are constantly being told what to/not to eat. What has changed over the last 100 years to our diet which has made us this way? Older generations were not as fat or as unhealthy as we are now. The worlds' national health services were not stretched to the extent they are now. Why can't we go back to a time where food was used as a fuel for the human body whilst also being enjoyed? After all, that's what food is for – a fuel for our bodies. We should be eating to live NOT living to eat. Unfortunately, that is exactly what most of us are doing – living to eat, and it is affecting us badly.

In this book, we are going to examine what we are eating at the moment, how it affects us and how we can change it. How to get ourselves slimmer, healthier and stay that way.

△△△

CONTENTS

1. THE CURRENT STATE OF WORLD DIET.   5
2. WHAT SHOULD WE BE EATING   7
3. WHAT IS IN OUR FOOD   11
4. WHAT FOODS SHOULD WE BE EATING   16
5. WEIGHT LOSS PLANS   19
6. SUMMARY   47

1. THE CURRENT STATE OF WORLD DIET.

With nearly 8 billion people on the planet with countless cultures and cuisines, it is hard to narrow down the perfect diet we should stick to. Over the generations, every part of the world adapted their diet to their local climate, job they were doing, temperature and what foods were available to them at the time and recipes were developed to provide maximum nutrition and where possible, flavour. To be fair, when you are hungry most things taste good! Older diets mostly evolved around vegetables, fruits and plants. Meat was eaten but far less regularly than is eaten nowadays. It was usually eaten on their rest day of the week (depending and where in the world you usually were). For example, in the United Kingdom it was a Sunday when a typical family would sit down for their Sunday 'roast'. Also, the food consumed in most diets was far less processed than it is now. There were less packaged products back then. Food was natural and whole, usually picked locally and then eaten within a few days. The human body was able to process these foods easily. Also, people were far more active in their jobs and in their way of living compared to now, which in turn helped the body to digest food better. People ate food to fuel their day.

What has changed since those days? In short. A LOT! Food

is still and always will be needed by humans for fuel. Without it for extended periods of time we cannot live without it. The food we are consuming has changed and the frequency of food consumption has changed too. Food has become big business and big businesses have the funds to manipulate what we eat, whether it is through advertising on TV, the Internet, social media, product placement in films and even to the extent of using scientific or medical research to convince us. Supermarkets constantly run promotions on products but usually they are on products which are enjoyed by most of us but are not great for our health or waistline, for example: cookies, chocolate, candy, bakery products etc. Also, the landscape of local highstreets has changed too. Whereas before there was a mix of local businesses supplying a wide range of products, now it is dominated by big shops/stores supplying a multitude of products which left a lot of shops unoccupied which in turn changed to fast food outlets. In order for these fast food shops to make a profit, the food they sell is highly processed to save on costly ingredients. These foods are NOT good for us. They do provide some sort of nutrition but the long-term effects of eating these foods are not good, as is plain to see by the state of our bodies in the modern age. These foods are harder to process, provide high calories, little useful nutritional value as well as a variety of harmful substitutes and food fillers to add flavour/texture to their food which remain in our bodies. We understand that people do enjoy fast food but it should be consumed very rarely and this does not mean once a day or week, it should be once a fortnight at a minimum. You read it right. Once a fortnight!

ΔΔΔ

2. WHAT SHOULD WE BE EATING

We live in a modern world, in a developed country so what should we all be eating? After all, everywhere we turn we are surrounded with choice. Good but mostly bad with a few choices in the middle. Well, that totally depends on what you would like your body to be like.

If you want to get big (fatter) then there are plenty of options out there. Deep fried, savoury products, pan pizzas', burgers, fried chicken, candy, doughnuts, fries etc. etc. the list is long and plentiful. These foods are readily available in every major town and city across the globe and most of the time is affordable. If you constantly eat these kinds of foods and don't exercise you will see yourself getting bigger, less fit, less mobile and visiting your doctor more and more often. Please don't fool yourself in thinking that you will are exception to this rule. It *will* happen! Also, the common mistake most people make, is to think 'it's ok, I'll have some fast food today and tomorrow I'll do better'. It's more than likely that you won't because the day after you will probably be thinking the same thing that you thought today.

If you want to stay healthy (recommended weight for

your height, age, gender), this can tie into losing weight too but we will continue with the weight loss in a moment. Staying at the correct weight for your height, gender and age depends on many factors to do with your own life, but as a general rule for a developed adult, the calorie intakes are:

Men 2500 calories per day

Women 2000 calories per day.

This can vary though depending on your own life circumstances and lifestyle.

Example 1: Female, 32 years old, 5'5" tall (167cm) with an office/desk job who walks most days for approximately 45 minutes and exercises for 1 hour, 3 times a week, will need 1900/2000 calories per day to maintain a healthy weight on non-workout days and 2000/2200 on workout days.

Example 2: Male, 40 years old, 5'11" tall (180cm) with a job involving light labour but exercises intensely 4-5 times a week, will need 2500/2700 calories per day to maintain his weight.

Both of these examples include a diet which is reliant on balanced home cooked foods which are diverse in nutrients. Eating whole food, fruits, vegetables. Lean meat is eaten but not every day. Exercising is a big factor in maintaining weight. It is well documented that healthy weight maintenance is 70% diet based (what you eat) and 30% exercise. If you don't exercise but eat healthily and consume calories consistent with what you expend, you will still maintain your weight, but your body will not be as good as it could be, for example, you will not be as toned or as athletically able as you could be. To maintain a healthy weight, the key is to:

- Eat healthy, whole foods,
- Reduce eating out frequently. Shops/restaurants/take-aways sell food and drink which makes them money. Not saying it is all bad, in fact there are some good choices but profit margins are their main agenda,

NOT your health or waistline.
- Increase consumption of water. Water is life. Water provides vital nutrients to our bodies which enable our organs to do the best job they can and water also helps the body to flush away the things it does not need. 2 liters or water a day is fine or more in warmer climates. This is a must!
- Exercise regularly. This does not mean you have to train like Arnold Schwarzenegger, it doesn't even mean you have to join a gym either even though it does help. It means incorporating physical activities in to your everyday life. Example: Getting to work. Why not walk there instead? If it's far, try walking half the journey or if you are using public transport try getting off 1 stop earlier than usual and walk 10 minutes. Do that to work and then again on the return journey is 20 minutes right there. Try walking to the shops, taking a stroll with a friend/partner or take the kids to the park, (Yours only. No one else's!!!). Cleaning your house/apartment is a calorie burner which gets you physical. If you don't join a gym or attend fitness classes, there is plenty of small changes you can make to be active which all add up to a big change. Best of all, you won't be feeling like you are working out and you are saving on gym membership fees too!
- If you get hungry between meal times having a small snack is fine. A piece of fruit, a handful of nuts, carrot batons etc. Just keep it small, keep it whole and only have it if hard to keep your hunger at bay until your next meal time. You don't want to be snacking regularly.
- Eat 3 main meals a day. Breakfast, Lunch and Dinner. You want your body to get used to eating at set times of the day so that you won't snack as much. There is a small exception to this rule though. Once every couple of weeks, skip a meal or if you can bear

it, try skipping 2 meals. There is a reason for this madness I promise! We have had access to plentiful amounts of food over the last century or so. Before this people would have to often skip a meal if food was not available but then replenish the calories on the next available meal. Fortunately, we are lucky that in todays' developed society that we have food available to us so we don't have the need to replenish the calories by skipping a meal but by skipping a meal in todays' diet promotes weight loss by increasing our metabolism in the short term. Our metabolism is a process which chemical reactions take place in our body which essentially take food and process it in to energy. The higher your metabolic rate, the more food your body can burn to create energy. It is a good idea to replace the skipped meal with lots of water. DO NOT skip meals frequently (i.e. skip meals once a day regularly) or go days without food. You want to keep your body and metabolic rate on its toes, you do not want to encourage fat storage. This is what your body will do when you go extended periods without having any food. The body will presume that food is not readily available when it is hungry and will try store excess fat from meals to burn when no food is available. This in itself is not a huge problem but a big problem will arise if you over eat on meal times then your body will have too much fat to convert to energy which will lead to WEIGHT GAIN. Obviously, this is not good and you will not want this.

∆∆∆

3. WHAT IS IN OUR FOOD

It is no coincidence that since we, I mean, businesses got involved in the food chain and the production of food – we as humans have become fat and unhealthy. There is money to be made at every stage of the food chain and you better believe that businesses are making it. Whether it is adding chemicals to aid the growing process of fruit and vegetables or adding drugs and unnatural additives to animal feed so that animals get bigger, faster. Food producing companies then take those manipulated products, then overly process them to maximise profits before selling them to restaurants/take-aways/supermarkets who then devise recipes which try to look as appetizing as possible and also as cheaply as possible. Some of the things which added in to food production is:

- Sodium Nitrate. A food colouring agent which aids in meat and poultry preservation.
- Propylene Glycol. Used for water absorption, anti-caking agent, texturing. Found in deodorants and Anti-Freeze.
- Silicone Dioxide. Used as an Anti-Caking agent. This is found in some natural food foods but in very small quantities such as leafy green vegetables, some peppers, brown rice and beetroot but is used

in food production on a larger scale which is not good for our bodies. Also found in Glass, Ceramics, Cement and at the beach in the form of Sand.
- Ammonium Sulfate. Classed as inorganic salt. Used as a dough enhancer for bread products and life extender. Can be used as a fertilizer.
- Cellulose. A.K.A. Wood pulp. Used as a thickener and food stabiliser. Cheaper to use than oil or flour. Found in Sauces, Ice Cream, Yogurt.
- Monosodium Glutamate (MSG). Used to add flavour to foods. Food standards agencies say this is safe to use in food but other research says it can cause brain malfunction and raise blood pressure.
- Dimethylpolysiloxane. Used as an Anti-Foaming and Anti-Caking agent. Makes oil last longer. Usually found in most restaurant and fast food outlet production methods. Found in Silly Putty, Breast implants, skin care products and some household products.
- Butylhydroquinone (TBHQ). Used as an Anti-Oxidant in fats and oils. Helps food last longer. Used in lighters, varnish, lacquer to name a few.

These are just a few of the things used in fast food and processed products we are surrounded by on our highstreets and supermarkets. Apart from being bad for our health these things are not easily processed by the body and when eaten regularly it is making us fat and sick. Although we have free choice to eat what we want, when we want to eat it, society has become used to eating these kinds of foods. Advertising even encourages us to do it. Some foods which we think is healthy and good for us, sometimes isn't. For example: Bran muffins, Low-Fat yogurts, salad dressings, Concentrated fruit juices, sports drinks, vegetable oils, chocolate covered fruit are just a very few examples. All of the above factors PLUS the fact the way most of us live our lives these days, with little to no exercise, is contributing to us being overweight and unhealthy.

There are now more overweight, obese and morbidly obese in the world than ever before and figures are set to only go in one direction – UP! Pharmaceutical companies are making an absolute fortune by supplying the sick for their illnesses, Illnesses which have come about because of their diet and their size. It is hard for overworked doctors to take the time to explain to each and every sick patient how to help get themselves better through better diet and exercise because there are so many patients who need this advice. It is easier to prescribe medicines and give out information leaflets which are rarely taken notice of. Pharmaceutical companies advise this and are more than happy for this to continue because the money will keep flowing in their direction.

There is a cycle of events which are designed to make big businesses money, to keep us spending but unfortunately it is at the expense of our health and also at the expense of our local health services. Please remember, Food producing companies want you to keep buying their products. Weight loss companies do not want everybody to lose weight and keep it off. Gyms do not want you to find alternate methods of working out. Pharmaceutical companies do not want you better in the long term. If everybody was fit and healthy, most of these companies would cease to exist. They wouldn't be making million or even billions of dollars that they are making now. It is down to you to get slimmer and healthier. This does not mean that you won't need help but it should not dictate your weight loss path. Let's have a look at how when we want to lose weight, we often get stuck in a couple of scenarios which keeps us in a continuous circle of bad weight management.

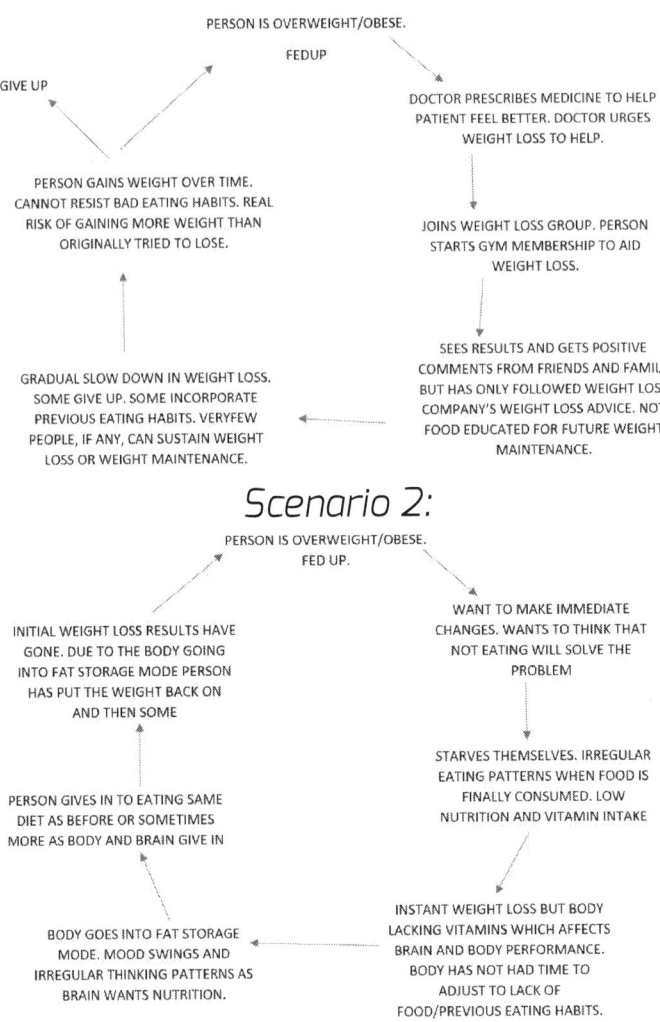

Remember, it doesn't matter what route you choose to lose weight, the likelyhood is that if you are overweight you will see weight loss results as soon as you begin to reduce your daily calorie consumption. The more overweight you are the more initial weight you will lose. This is where so many weight loss companies instill hope into people! You will lose and then gain. The trick is to lose the weight and then keep it off in you everyday life. Once at your target weight, it will be virtually impossible to stay at the exact same weight forever. Our bodies will always be fluctuating, the idea is that we have self awareness to regulate this ourselves. Example: A night out for a birthday meal with friends. 99% of the time, you won't find celery sticks and houmous on the menu! You indulge, as does everybody else with what takes your fancy, enjoy a few drinks and maybe some cake, after all it is a birthday! It is totally possible to intake your calories meant for the whole day in a matter of a few hours. This is on top of what you have eaten throughout the day. There is no way that the next morning you won't have put on a pound of two. This means that you will need to reduce your calorie intake by 200/300 over the next day or two to balance out. It won't be noticeable and your body will automatically make adjustments to use up the excess energy consumed on your night out. You can only make these adjustments yourself in what is good to eat and how much to consume. There is no magic pill. You want to break out of the 2 scenarios listed here previously. You want to forge your own scenario which look something like this:

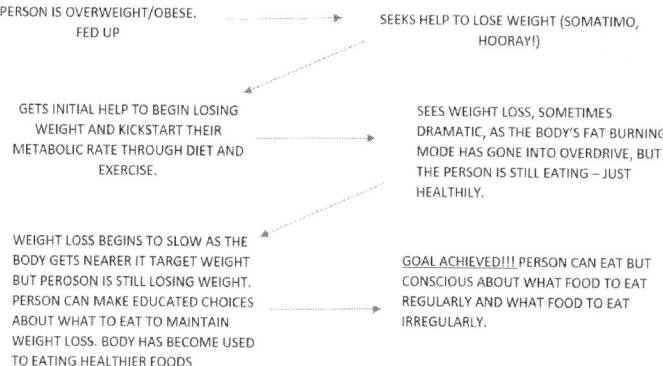

△△△

4. WHAT FOODS SHOULD WE BE EATING

This on one hand is a very easy question to answer and on the other hand rather hard. It's easy because there are many things that we should be eating to fulfil our nutrient requirements, foods that our bodies need and that we can enjoy but then that is hard to narrow down as we all live in different parts of the world where different things are available to us. We also all lead different lifestyles. Some have families, some people live alone. In an ideal scenario we would cook at home with organic ingredients that we bought ourselves and make our own meals for each day and take them with us to work too so we could eat when we were hungry. It's very rare that in today's society that we do this. Most of us grab something to eat when we are out so it is down to you to make informed choices once you have begun your weight loss journey. Let's have a look at what foods and drinks we should be eating regularly and what foods we should be mostly avoiding.

REGULAR ITEMS:
- WATER. 2 Liters per day minimum (6-8 glasses).
- VEGETABLES. Carrots, peas, broccoli, kale, spinach, beetroot, cucumber, onion, garlic, sweet potatoes, cabbage, zucchini (courgette), peppers, lettuce, tomatoes

(technically these are classed as fruit but grouped with most vegetables). These are a few examples. Keep it organic where possible.
- FRUITS. Apples, pears, plums, bananas, lemons, limes, grapefruit, oranges, mango, strawberries, avocados, berries, pineapple, pomegranate, melon, watermelon, olives are just a few.
- LEAN MEATS. Not everyday. Skin off always. Fat trimmed.
- WHOLE DAIRY ITEMS. Small quantities only. Always unsweetened. Whole milk and butter. Milk alternatives such as Soya, nut, coconut milk.
- NUTS. In small quantities and always unsalted.
- EXTRA VIRGIN OLIVE OIL AND COCONUT OIL. As little as possible only when cooking or olive oil as a dressing for salads.
- HERBS AND SPICES. For cooking and marinating.
- TEA. Free choice but try to enjoy without dairy where possible.
- COFFEE. Enjoy but again without dairy where possible and in limited quantities. 1-2 cups per day.

These foods and drinks are what you should be aiming to eat regularly. Aim for organic, low processed items. As with most things some are better than others. All have vital vitamins we need for function but some are also high in natural sugars and fat, sugars and fat that we need but in limited quantities. For example, you don't want to eat a lot of bananas or avocados everyday as they are vitamin rich but also fat and calorie dense too. Strawberries, plums, pears, apples are high in natural sugars so we don't want too consume too many everyday. You want your eating habits to be balanced. Too much of one thing is never good, no matter how healthy it seems to be.

IRREGULAR ITEMS:
- CANNED FRUITS AND VEGETABLES. Try to eat fresh where possible or frozen.

- CANDY. All processed and full of sugar.
- FATTY MEATS. Skin on, fat on.
- PROCESSED MEATS. Burgers, Hot dogs, Sausages, Salami, Corned beef.
- WHITE BREAD. Heavily processed.
- FRUIT JUICES. Better to eat the actual fruit. Fills the stomach and provides more vitamins thank just the sugar.
- PASTRIES, CAKES, COOKIES. None of these are healthy. Only fat and sugar are available in abundance.
- ENERGY DRINKS. Full of sugar and/or sweeteners. Get your energy through good eating and rest.
- FRIED/DEEP FRIED PRODUCTS. Chicken, fries, chips etc.
- BEER, DENSE ALCOHOLIC DRINKS.
- SODA.

These are types of foods and drinks to avoid consuming regularly. Some of the foods here are low in vitamins and good nutrition. Most are high in bad fats and sugars and will have a negative effect on your weight loss. More than likely, extended periods of eating these types of foods will lead to weight gain. Rule is, if it's processed, in a can, in a tub, in heavy packaging it will usually not be good for you. You want your food to be as organic as possible. We tend to check things in most aspects of our lives so why not spend a moment to check what you are putting into your body. After all, we only have one! Once you know what to look for in food, checking it will not take long to do and will eventually become 2nd nature so you won't even notice you are doing it.

$$\triangle\triangle\triangle$$

5. WEIGHT LOSS PLANS
(WHAT YOU REALLY CAME HERE FOR!)

I hear from so many people who are desperate to lose weight "Oh, if someone just told me what to eat then I would just eat that." Problem is, we are as a society DO get told what to eat. We are surrounded by so many different types of media with so much advertising that there is no way that we are not influenced in our choices of what to eat. Unfortunately for us, what we are told to eat is designed to make big companies money and keep us unhealthy, as mentioned in Scenario 1.

To help you to break this cycle and set you on the right path to hit your weight loss goals, below are 2, 28 day long weight loss plans. One for meat eaters and one for vegetarians. Then there are another 2 plans, again one for meat eaters and one for vegetarians but both are a little less strict to follow than the first two. These are labelled 'Higher calorie Intake'.

To be clear, none of the following plans are easy. There is no magic pill or spell can be cast which will make it easier. Will power and self organisation is required to complete. The higher calorie intake versions will be easier to stick to so if you think you might not stick to the stricter versions then it might be worth trying the latter 28 days plans first. You will see results with both but the harder plans will yield better results.

There are a few rules you must stick to in order to complete these plans as effectively as possible.

THE RULES:
1. Drink at least 2 liters of still water per day. Hunger is often confused with thirst. It is a good idea to have a glass of water before a meal. Black teas and black coffee is also permitted.
2. Try to prepare/cook the meals listed yourself. You will soon find it easy to stick to.
3. Keep the portions. Remember, just because the foods listed are good for you, you are trying to lose weight so calorie intake low. We will be aiming for a 1000-1300 calorie intake for most days.
4. Only eat what is stated on the plan.
5. There are usually 3 meals per day but there is no set time of day to eat them. You can plan when to eat every meal around your own lifestyle but you must plan to eat your final meal on each day no later than 3 hours before you would normally go to sleep.
6. You can swap meals per day. For example, swap dinner for lunch or vice versa but only what is listed. Do not swap daily meals with other days.
7. Be active (Important!). Calorie intake is low on the diet plan so trying to have a high intensity workout could be too strenuous for your body and could lead to you wanting to eat more than what is stated. You only need to be walking or doing light activities to be active. We are trying to change the metabolism of the body and this only happens through being active. Try going for a 20/30 minute walk AFTER every meal. Eat, wait 30 minutes, then be active. This is a must! If you can work out more a little more each day and are confident of not overeating after, then do it but please don't burn yourself out and end up in hospital. We want

your to lose weight and feel better, not worse!
8. Sleep! Yes we all do it anyway but sleep quality and length of sleep is important. You sleep should be uninterrupted and last between 6-7 hours only. Too much sleep leads to lethargic reactions and thinking. Not enough sleep leads to the body and brain wanting more food which leads to subconcious eating habits.
9. Keep busy. Extra time leads to extra eating if that is what you have been used to. When busy, most people tend to forget about eating.
10. When the 28 days are over you must increase your calorie intake to the recommended daily intake for your gender (2500 Men, 2000 Women) for at least a week. Do not diet in this week. Your body will need time to recover.
11. DO NOT ATTEMPT THIS DIET IF YOUR BMI IS LOWER THAN 22.

As with any diet or weight loss plan, if you unsure of any details above or have any concerns, please consult your Doctor.

MEAT EATERS 28 DAY PLAN:

WEEK 1

Day 1

B – 1 Slice dry toast with any tomato of your choice, raw or cooked (baby or cherry tomatoes limit 5)

L – Fresh fruit

D – 2 boiled or poached eggs. Salad with minimal dressing (olive oil, white vinegar, salt, pepper and lemon juice. Grapefruit for dessert.

Day 2

B – 1 boiled or poached egg. 1 whole grapefruit.

L – Grilled chicken with lemon juice. Small side salad with tomatoes.

D – Grilled steak (as lean as possible). Salad with minimal dressing and tomatoes.

Day 3

B - 1 boiled or poached egg. 1 whole grapefruit.

L – 1 Banana and any other fruit of choice.

D – 2 Grilled lamb chops with plenty of lemon juice, salad with dressing and tomatoes. Grapefruit for afters.

Day 4

B – 1 Slice of plain seeded toast.

L – 1 Banana and any other fresh fruit of choice.

D - 2 boiled or poached eggs. Salad with minimal dressing (olive oil, white vinegar, salt, pepper and lemon juice. Grapefruit for dessert.

Day 5

B – 1 Slice of plain seeded toast.

L – 1 Banana and any other fresh fruit of choice.

D – Grilled or oven baked fresh fish of your choice, lemon juice and salad.

Day 6

B – 1 Grapefruit.

L - 1 Banana and any other fresh fruit of choice.

D – Grilled chicken with lemon juice. Steamed or boiled broccoli and carrots.

Day 7

B – 2 scrambled eggs with tomatoes cooked any way.

L – 2 eggs cooked any way (except fried). With baby spinach.

D – Grilled steak (as lean as possible). Salad with minimal dressing and tomatoes.

Week 2

Day 1

B – 2 scrambled eggs with 2 rashers of grilled bacon (smoked or unsmoked).

1 Cup of coffee/tea with 1 sugar.

L – 1 natural yogurt.

D – 1 can of tuna (in water) and salad with tomatoes and dressing.

Day 2

B – 2 poached/scrambled eggs on 1 English muffin.

L - 1 Banana and any other fresh fruit of choice.

D – 1 Grilled steak with oven baked sweet potato with seasoning (whole of cut into fries)

Day 3

B – 1 Cup of coffee with 1 teaspoon of sugar.

L – 1 Handful (your handful, not the Hulk's!) plain or lightly salted nuts. Any is fine.

D – Grilled Pork loin chop with steam/boiled broccoli and carrots.

Day 4

B - 2 scrambled eggs with 2 rashers of grilled bacon (smoked or unsmoked). You can substitute bacon for smoked salmon.

L - 1 can tuna (in water), mixed with 1 tablespoon of light mayonnaise and ¼ cup of sweetcorn Sandwich in seeded brown bread.

D - 1 Handful (your handful, not the Hulk's!) plain or lightly salted nuts. Any is fine.

Day 5

B – (Nothing).

L – 2 Poached eggs and ½ avocado on 1 slice seeded brown toast.

D – 1 grilled fish of your choice with lemon juice and either boiled/steamed vegetables OR salad with tomatoes.

Day 6

B – 1 small natural yogurt.

L – 1 medium sized bowl of salad. Free choice.

D - Grilled steak with steamed/boiled broccoli and carrots.

Day 7

B – 2 Poached or scrambled eggs on 1 split English muffin served with 2 grilled bacon rashers OR 50g smoked salmon.

L – Grilled chicken breast with lemon juice and salad.

D – 2 toasted regular sized wholemeal pitta breads served with 150g Hummus.

WEEK 3

Day 1

B – 1 Cup of Coffee with 1 teaspoon of sugar.

L – 2 Boiled eggs, 1 regular tomato (5 cherry/baby), baby spinach.

D - Grilled steak (as lean as possible). Salad with minimal dressing and tomatoes.

Day 2

B - 1 Cup of Coffee with 1 teaspoon of sugar.

L - 250g ham, tomato (5 cherry/baby), 1 small natural yogurt.

D - Grilled steak (as lean as possible). Salad with minimal dressing and tomatoes.

Day 3

B - 1 Cup of Coffee with 1 teaspoon of sugar. 1 Slice of plain seeded toast.

L - 2 Boiled eggs with 1 slice of thick ham (2 thin) and salad with tomatoes. (Can incorporate all ingredients into a salad).

D - Boiled or steamed vegetables with seasoning. 1 item of fresh fruit for afters.

Day 4

B - 1 Cup of Coffee with 1 teaspoon of sugar. 1 Slice of plain seeded toast.

L - 1 Small natural yogurt and 1 glass of juice (orange or grapefruit).

D - 1 boiled egg and 250g cheese.

Day 5

B - 1 cup of coffee with 1 sugar.

L - 1 grilled/oven baked fresh fish of choice (1 small knob of butter permitted for cooking) served with boiled/steamed broccoli.

D - Grilled steak (as lean as possible). Salad with minimal dressing.

Day 6

B - 1 cup of coffee with 1 sugar.

L - 2 boiled eggs.

D - 1 Large chicken breast, grilled, with lemon juice and served with salad.

Day 7

B – 1 Cup of Coffee. No sugar. 1 Sweetener is permitted.

L – (Nothing)

D – 2 grilled lamb chops with lemon juice and salad.

Week 4

Day 1

B – 1 cup of coffee with 1 sugar.

L – 2 Boiled eggs with 1 tomato (5 baby/cherry) cooked any way and baby spinach.

D - Grilled steak (as lean as possible). Salad with minimal dressing.

Day 2

B - 1 cup of coffee with 1 sugar.

L - 250g ham, tomato (5 cherry/baby), 1 small natural yogurt.

D – 250g roasted beef (fresh or pre-sliced), salad with tomatoes and dressing.

Day 3

B - 1 Cup of Coffee with 1 teaspoon of sugar. 1 Slice of plain seeded toast.

L - 2 Boiled eggs with 1 slice of thick ham (2 thin) and salad with tomatoes. (Can incorporate all ingredients into a salad).

D - 1 Banana and any other fresh fruit of choice.

Day 4

B - 1 Cup of Coffee with 1 teaspoon of sugar. 1 Slice of plain seeded toast.

L - 1 Small natural yogurt and 1 glass of juice (orange or grapefruit).

D – 1 boiled egg and 250g cheese.

Day 5

B – 1 cup of coffee with 1 sugar.

L – 1 grilled/oven baked fresh fish of choice (1 small knob of butter permitted for cooking) served with boiled/steamed broccoli.

D - 250g roasted beef (fresh or pre-sliced), salad with tomatoes and dressing.

Day 6

B - 1 Cup of Coffee with 1 teaspoon of sugar. 1 Slice of plain seeded toast.

L – 2 Boiled eggs.

D - 1 Large chicken breast, grilled, with lemon juice and served with salad.

Day 7

B – 2 Scrambled or poached eggs on 1 English muffin.

L – (Nothing).

D - 1 Large chicken breast, grilled, with lemon juice and served with salad.

VEGETARIANS 28 DAY PLAN:

WEEK 1

Day 1

B – 1 Slice dry toast with any tomato of your choice, raw or cooked (baby or cherry tomatoes limit 5)

L – Fresh fruit

D – 2 boiled or poached eggs. Salad with minimal dressing (olive oil, white vinegar, salt, pepper and lemon juice. Grapefruit for dessert.

Day 2

B – 1 boiled or poached egg. 1 whole grapefruit.

L – 2 large portobello mushrooms with lemon juice. Small side salad with tomatoes.

D – 1 very large or 2 smaller cauliflower steak (prepared with your choice of seasoning). Salad with minimal dressing and tomatoes.

Day 3

B - 1 boiled or poached egg. 1 whole grapefruit.

L – 1 Banana and any other fruit of choice.

D – 2 Quorn burgers (do NOT fry) with plenty of lemon juice, salad with dressing and tomatoes. Grapefruit for afters.

Day 4

B – 1 Slice of plain seeded toast.

L – 1 Banana and any other fresh fruit of choice.

D - 2 boiled or poached eggs. Salad with minimal dressing (olive oil, white vinegar, salt, pepper and lemon juice. Grapefruit for dessert.

Day 5

B – 1 Slice of plain seeded toast.

L – 1 Banana and 1 other fresh fruit of choice.

D – Grilled or oven baked fresh fish of your choice OR Quorn fishless fillet (1 only), lemon juice and salad.

Day 6

B – 1 Grapefruit.

L - 1 Banana and any other fresh fruit of choice.

D – 2 portobello mushrooms with lemon juice and seasoning. Steamed or boiled broccoli and carrots.

Day 7

B – 2 scrambled eggs with tomatoes cooked any way.

L – 2 eggs cooked any way (except fried). With baby spinach.

D – 1 very large of 2 smaller cauliflower steaks (prepared with seasoning of your choice). Salad with minimal dressing and tomatoes.

Week 2

Day 1

B – 2 scrambled eggs on 1 seeded slice of bread or 1 English muffin. 1 Cup of coffee/tea with 1 sugar.

L – 1 natural yogurt.

D – 1 can of tuna (in water) and salad with tomatoes and dressing OR 1 large salad.

Day 2

B – 2 poached/scrambled eggs on 1 English muffin.

L - 1 Banana and 1 other fresh fruit of choice.

D – 1 very large of 2 smaller cauliflower steaks (prepared with seasoning of your choice). with oven baked sweet potato with seasoning (whole of cut into fries)

Day 3

B – 1 Cup of coffee with 1 teaspoon of sugar.

L – 1 Handful (your handful, not the Hulk's!) plain or lightly salted nuts. Any is fine.

D – A big bowl with steamed/boiled broccoli and carrots.

Day 4

B - 2 scrambled eggs.

L - ½ avocado, chopped and mixed with 1 tablespoon of light mayonnaise and tomato in a sandwich in seeded brown bread.

D - 1 Handful (your handful, not the Hulk's!) plain or lightly salted nuts. Any is fine.

Day 5

B - 1 whole grapefruit.

L - 2 Poached eggs and ½ avocado on 1 slice seeded brown toast.

D - 1 grilled fish OR 1 Quorn fishless fillet of your choice with lemon juice and either boiled/steamed vegetables OR salad with tomatoes.

Day 6

B - 1 small natural yogurt.

L - 1 medium sized bowl of salad. Free choice.

D - 2 Quorn burgers (NOT fried) with steamed/boiled broccoli and carrots.

Day 7

B - 2 Poached or scrambled eggs on 1 split English muffin served with 50g smoked salmon.

L - 2 large Portobello mushrooms with lemon juice and salad.

D - 2 toasted regular sized wholemeal pitta breads served with 150g Houmous.

WEEK 3

Day 1

B - 1 Cup of Coffee with 1 teaspoon of sugar. 1 grapefruit.

L - 2 Boiled eggs, 1 regular tomato (5 cherry/baby), baby spinach.

D - 1 very large of 2 smaller cauliflower steaks (prepared with seasoning of your choice). Salad with minimal dressing and tomatoes.

Day 2

B - 1 Cup of Coffee with 1 teaspoon of sugar.

L – 250g Quorn ham, tomato (5 cherry/baby), 1 small natural yogurt.

D – 2 Quorn burgers (NOT fried, only grilled) Salad with minimal dressing and tomatoes.

Day 3

B - 1 Cup of Coffee with 1 teaspoon of sugar. 1 Slice of plain seeded toast.

L – 2 Boiled eggs with 2 slices of Quorn ham and salad with tomatoes. (Can incorporate all ingredients into a salad).

D – Boiled or steamed vegetables with seasoning. 1 item of fresh fruit for afters.

Day 4

B - 1 Cup of Coffee with 1 teaspoon of sugar. 1 Slice of plain seeded toast.

L – 1 Small natural yogurt and 1 glass of juice (orange or grapefruit).

D – 1 boiled egg and 250g cheese.

Day 5

B – 1 grapefruit.

L – 1 grilled/oven baked fresh fish of choice (1 small knob of butter permitted for cooking) OR Quorn fishless fillets served with boiled/steamed broccoli.

D – Any Quorn alternative up to 170 calories per serving. 2 allowed. Salad with minimal dressing.

Day 6

B – 1 grapefruit. 1 coffee/tea with 1 sugar.

L – 2 boiled eggs with spinach.

D – 1 Large free choice salad. Cheese and avocado permitted.

Day 7
B – 1 Cup of Coffee. No sugar. 1 Sweetener is permitted.
L – 1 small natural yogurt.
D – 2 Quorn burgers (NOT fried) with lemon juice and salad.

Week 4
Day 1
B – 1 cup of coffee with 1 sugar.
L – 2 Boiled eggs with 1 tomato (5 baby/cherry) cooked any way and baby spinach.
D – 2 Portobello mushrooms with lemon juice. Salad with minimal dressing.

Day 2
B - 1 cup of coffee with 1 sugar.
L – 200g Quorn ham slices, tomato (5 cherry/baby), 1 small natural yogurt.
D – 1 Avocado salad with tomatoes and dressing.

Day 3
B - 1 Cup of Coffee with 1 teaspoon of sugar. 1 Slice of plain seeded toast.
L - 2 Boiled eggs with 2 slices of Quorn ham and salad with tomatoes. (Can incorporate all ingredients into a salad).
D - 1 Banana and any other fresh fruit of choice.

Day 4
B - 1 Cup of Coffee with 1 teaspoon of sugar. 1 Slice of plain seeded toast.
L - 1 Small natural yogurt and 1 glass of juice (orange or grapefruit).

D – 1 boiled egg and 250g cheese.

Day 5

B – 1 grapefruit.

L – 1 grilled/oven baked fresh fish of choice (1 small knob of butter permitted for cooking) OR Quorn fishless fillet served with boiled/steamed broccoli.

D – 1 Avocado salad with tomatoes and dressing.

Day 6

B - 1 Cup of Coffee with 1 teaspoon of sugar. 1 Slice of plain seeded toast.

L – 2 Boiled eggs.

D - 1 very large of 2 smaller cauliflower steaks (prepared with seasoning of your choice) and served with salad.

Day 7

B – 2 Scrambled or poached eggs on 1 English muffin.

L – (Nothing).

D – 200g Quorn roasted beef with lemon juice and broccoli and carrots.

MEAT EATERS 28 DAY PLAN (HIGHER CALORIE INTAKE)

WEEK 1

Day 1

B – 1 small pot of natural yogurt or 2 tablespoons if using a larger pot.

L – As much fresh fruit as you want of your choice.

D – 2 boiled or poached eggs. Salad with minimal dressing (olive oil, white vinegar, salt, pepper and lemon juice. Grapefruit for dessert.

Day 2

B – 2 boiled or poached eggs on 1 toast or English muffin. 1 whole grapefruit.

L – Grilled chicken with lemon juice. Small side salad with tomatoes.

D – Grilled steak (as lean as possible). Salad with minimal dressing and tomatoes.

Day 3

B – 2 boiled or poached egg on 1 toast or English muffin. 1 whole grapefruit.

L – As much fresh fruit as you want of your choice.

D – 2 Grilled lamb chops with plenty of lemon juice, salad with dressing and tomatoes. Grapefruit for afters.

Day 4

B – 2 Slices of plain seeded toast.

L – As much fresh fruit as you want of your choice.

D – Grilled chicken Salad with minimal dressing (olive oil, white vinegar, salt, pepper and lemon juice. Can add avocado too. Grapefruit for dessert.

Day 5

B – 2 Slices of plain seeded toast.

L – As much fresh fruit as you want of your choice.

D – Grilled or oven baked fresh fish of your choice, lemon juice and salad of your choice.

Day 6

B – 1 small natural yogurt or 2 tablespoons if using a larger pot.

L - As much fresh fruit as you want of your choice.

D – Grilled chicken with lemon juice. Steamed or boiled broccoli and carrots.

Day 7

B – 2 scrambled eggs with tomatoes cooked any way.

L – Grilled chicken and avocado sandwich on seeded bread or wrap.

D - Grilled steak (as lean as possible). Salad with minimal dressing and tomatoes.

Week 2

Day 1

B – 2 scrambled eggs with 2 rashers of grilled bacon (smoked or unsmoked).

1 Cup of coffee/tea with 1 sugar.

L – 1 natural yogurt.

D – 1 can of tuna and salad with tomatoes and dressing.

Day 2

B – 2 poached/scrambled eggs on 1 English muffin.

L - As much fresh fruit as you want of your choice.

D – 1 Grilled steak with oven baked sweet potato with seasoning (whole of cut into fries)

Day 3

B – 2 plain toast (seeded). 1 Cup of coffee with 1 teaspoon of sugar.

L – 1 Handful (your handful, not the Hulk's!) plain or lightly salted nuts. Any is fine.

D – Grilled Pork loin chop with steam/boiled broccoli and carrots.

Day 4

B - 2 scrambled eggs with 2 rashers of grilled bacon (smoked or unsmoked). You can substitute bacon for smoked salmon.

L – 1 can tuna (in water), mixed with 1 tablespoon of light mayonnaise and ¼ cup of sweetcorn Sandwich in seeded brown bread.

D - 1 Handful (your handful, not the Hulk's!) plain or lightly salted nuts. Any is fine.

Day 5

B – 1 natural yogurt or 2 tablespoons if using a larger pot.

L – 2 Poached eggs and ½ avocado on 1 slice seeded brown toast.

D – 1 grilled fish of your choice with lemon juice and either boiled/steamed vegetables OR salad with tomatoes.

Day 6

B – 1 natural yogurt.

L – 1 medium sized bowl of salad. Free choice.

D – Free choice! Take aways included. Keep portion small/medium.

Day 7

B – 2 Poached or scrambled eggs on 1 split English muffin. Can also have 2 rashers of grilled bacon.

L – Grilled chicken breast with lemon juice and salad.

D – 2 toasted regular sized wholemeal pitta breads served with 150g Hummus.

WEEK 3

Day 1

B – 1 whole grapefruit. 1 Cup of Coffee with 1 teaspoon of sugar.

L – 2 Boiled eggs on seeded toast or 1 split English muffin.

D - Grilled steak (as lean as possible). Salad with minimal dressing and tomatoes.

Day 2

B - 1 Cup of Coffee with 1 teaspoon of sugar.

L - Ham and tomato sandwich on seeded bread, 1 small natural yogurt.

D - Grilled steak (as lean as possible). Salad with minimal dressing and tomatoes.

Day 3

B - 1 Cup of Coffee with 1 teaspoon of sugar. 1 Slice of plain seeded toast.

L - 2 Boiled eggs with 1 slice of thick ham (2 thin) and salad with tomatoes. (Can incorporate all ingredients into a salad).

D - Large bowl of boiled or steamed vegetables with seasoning. Fresh fruit for afters.

Day 4

B - 1 Cup of Coffee with 1 teaspoon of sugar. 2 Slices of plain seeded toast.

L - 1 Small natural yogurt and 1 piece of fruit.

D - 2 egg omelette with free choice toppings

Day 5

B - 1 handful of nuts (free choice). 1 cup of coffee with 1 sugar.

L - 1 grilled/oven baked fresh fish of choice (1 small knob of butter permitted for cooking) served with boiled/steamed broccoli.

D - Grilled steak (as lean as possible). Salad with minimal dressing.

Day 6

B - 2 boiled eggs with toast soldiers. 1 cup of coffee with 1 sugar.

L - 1 handful of nuts and a piece of fruit (free choice).

D – 1 Large chicken breast, grilled, with lemon juice and served with salad.

Day 7

B – 1 Cup of Coffee. No sugar. 1 Sweetener is permitted.

L – (Nothing)

D – 2 grilled lamb chops with lemon juice and salad.

Week 4

Day 1

B – 1 cup of coffee with 1 sugar and 1 slice of plain toast.

L – 2 scrambled eggs with baby spinach. 1 piece of fruit.

D - Grilled steak (as lean as possible). Salad with minimal dressing.

Day 2

B - 1 cup of coffee with 1 sugar. 1 small natural yogurt.

L – Ham and tomato sandwich on seeded bread or wrap.

D – Steak salad with tomatoes and dressing.

Day 3

B - 1 Cup of Coffee with 1 teaspoon of sugar. 1 Slice of plain seeded toast.

L - 2 Boiled eggs with 1 slice of thick ham (2 thin) and salad with tomatoes. (Can incorporate all ingredients into a salad).

D – As much fresh fruit as you want. Try to include a banana.

Day 4

B - 1 Cup of Coffee with 1 teaspoon of sugar. 1 Slice of plain seeded toast.

L - 1 Small natural yogurt and 1 glass of juice (orange or grapefruit).

D – 1 boiled egg and 250g cheese.

Day 5

B – 1 cup of coffee with 1 sugar and 1 plain slice of toast.

L – 1 grilled/oven baked fresh fish of choice (1 small knob of butter permitted for cooking) served with boiled/steamed broccoli.

D – Steak salad with tomatoes and dressing.

Day 6

B - 1 Cup of Coffee with 1 teaspoon of sugar.

L – 2 Boiled or scrambled eggs on 2 toast.

D - 1 Large chicken breast, grilled, with lemon juice and served with salad.

Day 7

B – 2 Scrambled or poached eggs on 1 English muffin.

L – Fresh fruit of your choice.

D - 1 Large chicken breast, grilled, with lemon juice and served with salad.

VEGETARIANS 28 DAY PLAN (HIGHER CALORIE INTAKE):

WEEK 1

Day 1

B – 1 Natural yogurt or 2 tablespoons if using a larger pot.

L – Any amount of fresh fruit of your choice.

D – 2 boiled or poached eggs. Salad with minimal dressing (olive oil, white vinegar, salt, pepper and lemon juice. Grapefruit for dessert.

Day 2

B – 2 boiled or poached eggs on 1 toast or English muffin. 1 whole grapefruit.

L – 2 large portobello mushrooms with lemon juice and another topping of your choice. Small side salad with tomatoes.

D – 1 very large or 2 smaller cauliflower steak (prepared with your choice of seasoning). Salad with minimal dressing and tomatoes.

Day 3

B – 2 boiled or poached egg on 1 toast or English muffin. 1 whole grapefruit.

L – As much fresh fruit as you want of your choice.

D – 2 Quorn burgers (do NOT fry) with plenty of lemon juice, salad with dressing and tomatoes. Grapefruit for afters.

Day 4

B – 2 Slices of plain seeded toast.

L – As much fresh fruit as you want of your choice.

D – 2 egg omelette with free choice of topping but try to include a veg topping. Grapefruit for dessert.

Day 5

B – 2 Slices of plain seeded toast.

L – As much fresh fruit as you want of your choice.

D – Grilled or oven baked fresh fish of your choice OR Quorn fishless fillet (1 only), lemon juice and salad.

Day 6

B – 1 small natural yogurt or 2 tablespoons if using a larger pot.

L – As much fresh fruit as you want of your choice.

D – 2 portobello mushrooms with lemon juice and seasoning. Steamed or boiled broccoli and carrots.

Day 7

B – 2 scrambled eggs with tomatoes cooked any way.

L – Avocado, tomato and spinach sandwich on seeded bread or panini. Toasted if you prefer.

D – 1 very large of 2 smaller cauliflower steaks (prepared with seasoning of your choice). Salad with minimal dressing and tomatoes.

Week 2

Day 1

B – 2 scrambled eggs or poached on 1 English muffin with 1 Cup of coffee/tea with 1 sugar.

L – 1 natural yogurt or 2 tablespoons if using a larger pot.

D – 1 can of tuna (in water) and salad with tomatoes and dressing OR 1 large salad.

Day 2

B – 2 poached/scrambled eggs on 1 English muffin.

L – As much fresh fruit as you want of your choice.

D – 1 very large of 2 smaller cauliflower steaks (prepared with seasoning of your choice). with oven baked sweet potato with seasoning (whole of cut into fries)

Day 3

B – 2 plain toast (seeded). 1 Cup of coffee with 1 teaspoon of sugar.

L – 1 Handful (your handful, not the Hulk's!) plain or lightly salted nuts. Any is fine.

D – A big bowl with steamed/boiled broccoli and carrots.

Day 4

B – 2 scrambled eggs on 1 English muffin. You can add a small side of your choice if you like.

L – 1 can tuna (in water), mixed with 1 tablespoon of light mayonnaise and ¼ cup of sweetcorn Sandwich in seeded brown bread.

D – 1 Handful (your handful, not the Hulk's!) plain or lightly salted nuts. Any is fine.

Day 5

B – 1 natural yogurt or 2 tablespoons if using a larger pot.

L – 2 Poached eggs and ½ avocado on 1 slice seeded brown toast.

D – 1 grilled fish OR 1 Quorn fishless fillet of your choice with lemon juice and either boiled/steamed vegetables OR salad with tomatoes.

Day 6

B – 1 small natural yogurt or 2 tablespoons if using a larger pot.

L – 1 medium sized bowl of salad. Free choice.

D – Free choice! Take aways included. Keep portion small/medium.

Day 7

B – 2 Poached or scrambled eggs on 1 split English muffin. Can have 50g of smoked salmon if you wish.

L – 2 large Portobello mushrooms with lemon juice and salad. Stuff the mushrooms if you wish with a small filling of your choice.

D – 2 toasted regular sized wholemeal pitta breads served with 150g Hummus.

WEEK 3

Day 1

B – 1 Cup of Coffee with 1 teaspoon of sugar. 1 grapefruit.

L – 2 Boiled or scrambled eggs on seeded toast or 1 split English muffin.

D – 1 very large of 2 smaller cauliflower steaks (prepared with seasoning of your choice). Salad with minimal dressing and tomatoes.

Day 2

B – 1 Cup of Coffee with 1 teaspoon of sugar.

L – Free choice sandwich on seeded bread and 1 natural yogurt.

D – 2 Quorn burgers (NOT fried, only grilled) Salad with minimal dressing and tomatoes.

Day 3

B – 1 Cup of Coffee with 1 teaspoon of sugar. 1 Slice of plain seeded toast.

L – 2 Boiled eggs and salad with tomatoes. (Can incorporate all ingredients into a salad). You can add a small amount of cheese if you wish.

D – Boiled or steamed vegetables with seasoning. 1 item of fresh fruit for afters.

Day 4

B – 1 Cup of Coffee with 1 teaspoon of sugar. 2 Slices of plain seeded toast.

L – 1 Small natural yogurt and 1 piece of fruit of your choice.

D – 2 egg omelette with cheese, mushroom and bell pepper.

Day 5

B – 1 handful of nuts (free choice). 1 cup of coffee with 1 sugar.

L – 1 grilled/oven baked fresh fish of choice (1 small knob of butter permitted for cooking) OR Quorn fishless fillets served with boiled/steamed broccoli.

D – Any Quorn alternative. 1 portion. Salad with minimal dressing.

Day 6

B – 2 boiled eggs with toast soldiers. 1 cup of coffee with 1 sugar.

L – 1 handful of nuts and a piece of fruit (free choice).

D – 1 Large free choice salad. Cheese and avocado permitted or feel free to include a Quorn product of your choice too if you are not including cheese.

<u>Day 7</u>

B – 1 Cup of Coffee. No sugar. 1 Sweetener is permitted.

L – 1 small natural yogurt or 2 tablespoons if using a larger pot.

D – 2 Quorn burgers (NOT fried) with lemon juice and salad.

<u>Week 4</u>

<u>Day 1</u>

B – 1 cup of coffee with 1 sugar.

L – 2 Boiled or scrambled eggs with 1 tomato (5 baby/cherry) cooked any way and baby spinach. 1 piece of fruit.

D – 2 Portobello mushrooms with lemon juice. Salad with minimal dressing.

<u>Day 2</u>

B - 1 cup of coffee with 1 sugar. 1 small natural yogurt.

L – Quorn ham slices and tomato sandwich on seeded bread or wrap.

D – Free choice large salad with 1 added Quorn product of your choice.

<u>Day 3</u>

B - 1 Cup of Coffee with 1 teaspoon of sugar. 1 Slice of plain seeded toast.

L - 2 Boiled eggs with 2 slices of Quorn ham and salad with tomatoes. (Can incorporate all ingredients into a salad).

D - As much fresh fruit as you want. Try to include a banana if possible.

Day 4

B - 1 Cup of Coffee with 1 teaspoon of sugar. 1 Slice of plain seeded toast.

L - 1 Small natural yogurt and 1 glass of juice (orange or grapefruit).

D – 1 boiled egg and 250g cheese.

Day 5

B – 1 cup of coffee with 1 sugar and 1 plain slice of toast.

L – 1 grilled/oven baked fresh fish of choice (1 small knob of butter permitted for cooking) OR Quorn fishless fillet served with boiled/steamed broccoli.

D – Free choice salad with avocado and dressing.

Day 6

B - 1 Cup of Coffee with 1 teaspoon of sugar. 1 Slice of plain seeded toast.

L – 2 Boiled or scrambled eggs on toast.

D - 1 very large of 2 smaller cauliflower steaks (prepared with seasoning of your choice) and served with salad.

Day 7

B – 2 Scrambled or poached eggs on 1 English muffin.

L – Fresh fruit of your choice.

D – 200g Quorn roasted beef with lemon juice and broccoli and carrots.

You should expect to lose anywhere between 20 pounds (1.4 stone, 9 KG) and 50 pounds (3.6 stone, 22.6 KG) in 28 days. This is totally dependent on your starting weight, daily activity and portion control throughout the 28 days. As mentioned before, these are not easy to follow but each plan only lasts 28 days so if you can stick to it, please do so. If you feel you cannot follow it properly or begin to not feel well please STOP.

AGAIN, DO NOT ATTEMPT THIS DIET IF YOUR BMI IS LOWER THAN 22.

6. SUMMARY

No one is perfect. We all slip up in most areas of our lives at some point but it is important to remember that slipping up on your weight loss journey is pretty much a given – we are human after all. Do not let a small slip up affect your goal or dishearten you so that you end up quitting. The body is an amazing thing. It will readjust itself many times over, so if you slip get back on the horse and carry on.

Will power is needed in many areas of our lives and it is no different here. If you don't want to lose weight whole heartedly then it is inevitable that you will fail. You must want to lose weight in order for it to happen. Our minds are powerful things and it is amazing what positive and wilful thinking can have on the body. It has been said that it is possible to think yourself slim. Although that statement is a bit extreme, there is no doubt that positive thinking will have a positive effect on your body and together with a good diet and exercise you will have no problem hitting your weight loss goals. Why wait? Do it today!

For further information, or for your bespoke weight loss plan, Please visit us at WWW.TASMICHAEL.COM

Copyright 2019. Tas Michael. All rights reserved.

Printed in Great Britain
by Amazon